MW00511485

# Easy Ketogenic Diet for Beginners 2021

## The Complete Keto Diet Cookbook to Lose Weight Without Giving Up your Favorite Dishes

**Allison Rivera**

© Copyright 2021 - Allison Rivera - All rights reserved.

The content contained within this book may not be reproduced, duplicated or transmitted without direct written permission from the author or the publisher.

Under no circumstances will any blame or legal responsibility be held against the publisher, or author, for any damages, reparation, or monetary loss due to the information contained within this book. Either directly or indirectly.

**Legal Notice:**

This book is copyright protected. This book is only for personal use. You cannot amend, distribute, sell, use, quote or paraphrase any part, or the content within this book, without the consent of the author or publisher.

**Disclaimer Notice:**

Please note the information contained within this document is for educational and entertainment purposes only. All effort has been executed to present accurate, up to date, and reliable, complete information. No warranties of any kind are declared or implied. Readers acknowledge that the author is not engaging in the rendering of legal, financial, medical or professional advice. The content within this book has been derived from various sources. Please consult a licensed professional before attempting any techniques outlined in this book.

By reading this document, the reader agrees that under no circumstances is the author responsible for any losses, direct or indirect, which are incurred as a result of the use of information contained within this document, including, but not limited to, — errors, omissions, or inaccuracies

# Table of Content

# SMOOTHIES & BREAKFAST

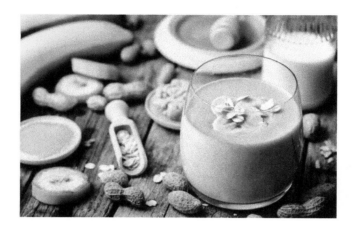

# Carrot Chaffle Cake

Preparation Time: 15 minutes Cooking Time: 24 minutes
Servings: 6

**Ingredients:**

- 1 egg, beaten

- 2 tablespoons melted butter

- ½ cup carrot, shredded

- ¾ cup almond flour

- 1 teaspoon baking powder

- 2 tablespoons heavy whipping cream

- 2 tablespoons sweetener

- 1 tablespoon walnuts, chopped

- 1 teaspoon pumpkin spice
- 2 teaspoons cinnamon

**Directions:**

1. Preheat your waffle maker.

2. In a large bowl, combine all the ingredients.

3. Pour some of the mixture into the waffle maker.

4. Close and cook for 4 minutes.

5. Repeat steps until all the remaining batter has been used.

Nutrition: Calories 294 Total Fat 26.7g Saturated Fat 12g Cholesterol 133mg Sodium 144mg Potassium 421mg Total Carbohydrate 11.6g Dietary Fiber 4.5g Protein 6.8g Total Sugars 1.7g

# Blueberry Chaffles

Preparation Time: 10 minutes Cooking Time: 28 minutes Servings: 4

**Ingredients:**

- **1 egg, beaten**

- **½ cup finely grated mozzarella cheese**

- **1 tbsp cream cheese, softened**

- **1 tbsp sugar-free maple syrup**
  + extra for topping

- **½ cup blueberries**

- **¼ tsp vanilla extract**

# Whole Wheat Pecan Chaffles

Serving: 8

Preparation Time: 10 minutes Cooking Time: 20 minutes

Ingredients

- 2 cups whole wheat pastry flour

- 2 tablespoons sugar

- 3 teaspoons baking powder

- 1/2 teaspoon salt

- 1/2 cup mozzarella cheese, shredded
- 2 large eggs, separated

- 1-3/4 cups fat-free milk

- 1/4 cup canola oil

- 1/2 cup chopped pecans

Direction

1. **Preheat waffle maker. Whisk together first four ingredients. In another bowl, whisk together egg yolks, milk and oil; add to flour mixture, stirring just until moistened. In a clean bowl, beat egg whites on medium speed until stiff but not dry. Add mozzarella cheese and stir well.**

2. **Fold into batter. Bake chaffles according to manufacturer's directions until golden brown, sprinkling batter with pecans after pouring. Freeze option: Cool chaffles on wire racks. Freeze between layers of waxed paper in a resealable plastic freezer bag. Reheat chaffles in a toaster or toaster oven on medium setting.**

Nutrition: Calories: 241 calories Total Fat: 14g Cholesterol: 48mg Sodium: 338mg Total Carbohydrate: 24g Protein: 7g Fiber: 3g

# Wednesday
# Chaffles

Serving: 24

Preparation Time: 10 minutes Cooking Time: 55 minutes

Ingredients

- **cooking spray**

- **8 eggs, beaten**

- **7 cups water**

- **1 cup canola oil**

- **1 cup unsweetened applesauce**

- **4 teaspoons vanilla extract**

- **4 cups whole wheat pastry flour**

- **2 cups dry milk powder**

- **1/2 cup mozzarella cheese, shredded**

- **2 cups flax seed meal**

- **1 cup wheat germ**

- **1 cup all-purpose flour**

- 1/4 cup baking powder

- 4 teaspoons baking powder

- 1/4 cup white sugar

- 1 tablespoon ground cinnamon

- 1 teaspoon salt

Direction

1. Spray a waffle iron with cooking spray and preheat according to manufacturer's instructions.

2. Beat eggs, water, canola oil, applesauce, and vanilla extract in a large bowl thoroughly combined. Add mozzarella cheese and stir well.

3. Whisk whole wheat pastry flour, dry milk powder, flax seed meal, wheat germ, all-purpose flour, 1/4 cup plus 4 teaspoons baking powder, sugar, cinnamon, and salt in a separate large bowl until thoroughly combined. Mix dry ingredients into wet ingredients 1 cup at a time to make a smooth batter.

4. Ladle 1/2 cup batter, or amount recommended by manufacturer, into preheated waffle iron; close lid and cook waffle until crisp and browned, 3 to 5 minutes. Repeat with remaining batter.

**Nutrition:**

Calories: 313 calories Total Fat: 15.9
g Cholesterol: 64 mg Sodium: 506 mg Total Carbohydrate: 33.4 g
Protein: 11.8 g

**Directions:**

1.  **Preheat the waffle iron.**

2.  **Mix all the ingredients in a**
    medium bowl.

3.  **Open the iron and pour in a quarter of
    the mixture. Close and cook until crispy,
    6 minutes.**

4.  **Remove the chaffle onto a plate and
    make 3 more with the remaining
    ingredients.**

5.  **Cut each chaffle into wedges, plate, allow
    cooling and serve.**

Nutrition: Calories 136 Fats 9.45g Carbs 3.69g Net Carbs 3.69g Protein 8.5g

# Healthy Green

# Smoothie

Preparation Time: 5 minutes Cooking Time: 5 minutes

Serve: 2

## Ingredients:

- 1 cup avocado
- 1/2 lemon, peeled
- 1 cucumber, peeled
- 1 tsp ginger, peeled
- 1/2 cup cilantro
- 1 cup baby spinach
- 1 cup of water

## Directions:

Add all ingredients into the blender and blend until smooth. Serve and enjoy.

## Nutritional Value (Amount per Serving):

Calories 179
Fat 14.5 g
Carbohydrates 13.1 g
Sugar 3 g
Protein 3 g

Cholesterol 0 mg

**Directions:**

1. Preheat the waffle iron.

2. In a medium bowl, mix all the ingredients.

3. Open the iron, lightly grease with cooking spray and pour in a quarter of the mixture.

4. Close the iron and cook until golden brown and crispy, 7 minutes.

5. Remove the chaffle onto a plate and set aside.

6. Make the remaining chaffles with the remaining mixture.

7. Drizzle the chaffles with maple syrup and serve afterward.

Nutrition: Calories 137 Fats 9.07g Carbs 4.02g Net Carbs 3.42g Protein 9.59g

# Chaffle Cannoli

Preparation Time: 15 minutes Cooking Time: 28 minutes Servings: 4

**Ingredients:**
**For the chaffles:**

- **1 large egg**

- **1 egg yolk**

- **3 tbsp butter, melted**

- **1 tbso swerve confectioner's**

- **1 cup finely grated Parmesan cheese**

- **2 tbsp finely grated**
  mozzarella cheese

**For the cannoli filling:**

- **½ cup ricotta cheese**

- **2 tbsp swerve confectioner's sugar**

- **1 tsp vanilla extract**

- **2 tbsp unsweetened chocolate chips for garnishing**

**Directions:**

2. Preheat the waffle iron.

3. Meanwhile, in a medium bowl, mix all the ingredients for the chaffles.

4. Open the iron, pour in a quarter of the mixture, cover, and cook until crispy, 7 minutes.

5. Remove the chaffle onto a plate and make 3 more with the remaining batter.

6. Meanwhile, for the cannoli filling:

7. Beat the ricotta cheese and swerve confectioner's sugar until smooth. Mix in the vanilla.

8. On each chaffle, spread some of the filling and wrap over.

9. Garnish the creamy ends with some chocolate chips.

10. Serve immediately.

Nutrition: Calories 308 Fats 25.05g Carbs 5.17g Net Carbs 5.17g Protein 15.18g

# Nutter Butter
# Chaffles

Preparation Time: 15 minutes Cooking Time: 14 minutes Servings: 2

**Ingredients:**
**For the chaffles:**

- **2 tbsp sugar-free peanut butter powder**

- **2 tbsp maple (sugar-free) syrup**

- **1 egg, beaten**

- **¼ cup finely grated mozzarella cheese**

- **¼ tsp baking powder**

- **¼ tsp almond butter**

- **¼ tsp peanut butter extract**

- **1 tbsp softened cream cheese**

**For the frosting:**

- **½ cup almond flour**

- **1 cup peanut butter**

- 3 tbsp almond milk

- ½ tsp vanilla extract

- ½ cup maple (sugar-free) syrup

**Directions:**

2. Preheat the waffle iron.

3. Meanwhile, in a medium
   bowl, mix all the ingredients until smooth.

4. Open the iron and pour in half of the mixture.

5. Close the iron and cook until crispy, 6 to 7 minutes.

6. Remove the chaffle onto a plate and set aside.

7. Make a second chaffle with the remaining batter.

8. While the chaffles cool, make the frosting.

9. Pour the almond flour in a medium saucepan and stir-fry over medium heat until golden.

10. Transfer the almond flour to a blender

**and top with the remaining frosting ingredients. Process until smooth.**

**11. 1Spread the frosting on the chaffles and serve afterward.**

Nutrition: Calories 239 Fats 15.48g Carbs 17.42g Net Carbs 15.92g Protein 7.52g

# Roasted Pepper

# Chicken

Preparation Time: 10 minutes Cooking Time: 15 minutes Serve: 4

**Ingredients:**

- 4 chicken breasts, skinless and boneless
- 1 1/2 tsp Italian seasoning
- 2/3 cup red peppers, roasted and chopped
- 3/4 cup heavy cream
- 3 garlic cloves, minced
- 4 tbsp olive oil
- 1/2 tsp salt

**Directions:**

1. Add pepper, garlic, oil, 1 teaspoon Italian seasoning, pepper, and salt into the blender and blend until smooth.
2. Season chicken with remaining seasoning and cook in a pan over medium heat for 7-8 minutes on each side.
3. Transfer chicken to a plate.
4. Pour red pepper mixture into the pan and cook for 2 minutes.
5. Add heavy cream and stir well.
6. Return chicken to the pan stir well to coat with sauce.
7. Serve and enjoy.

## Nutritional Value (Amount per Serving):

Calories 520

Fat 37 g

Carbohydrates 5 g

Sugar 2 g

Protein 42 g

Cholesterol 10 mg

# SEAFOOD & FISH RECIPES

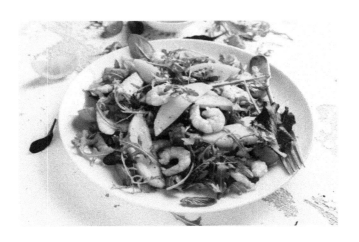

# Shrimp & Broccoli

Preparation Time: 10 minutes Cooking Time: 7

minutes

Serve: 2

## Ingredients:

- 1/2 lb shrimp
- 1 tsp fresh lemon juice
- 2 tbsp butter
- 2 garlic cloves, minced
- 1 cup broccoli florets
- Salt

## Directions:

- Melt butter in a pan over medium heat.
- Add garlic and broccoli to pan and cook for 3-4 minutes.
- Add shrimp and cook for 3-4 minutes.
- Add lemon juice and salt and stir well.
- Serve and enjoy.

## Nutritional Value (Amount per Serving):

Calories 257

Fat 13 g

Carbohydrates 6 g

Sugar 0.9 g

Protein 27 g

Cholesterol 269 mg

# Smooth Broccoli Cauliflower Mashed

Preparation Time: 10 minutes Cooking Time: 10 minutes Serve: 4

## Ingredients:

- 2 cups cauliflower florets
- 2 cups broccoli florets
- 2 garlic cloves, peeled
- ¼ tsp onion powder
- 1 tbsp olive oil
- 1/2 tsp pepper
- 1/2 tsp salt

## Directions:

1. Heat olive oil in a pan over medium heat.
2. Add cauliflower, broccoli, and salt in a pan and sauté until softened.
3. Transfer vegetables and garlic to the food processor and process until smooth.
4. Season with onion powder, pepper and salt.
5. Serve and enjoy.

## Nutritional Value (Amount per Serving):

Calories 60

Fat 3 g

Carbohydrates 6 g

Sugar 2 g

Protein 2 g

Cholesterol 0 mg

# PORK, BEEF & LAMB RECIPES

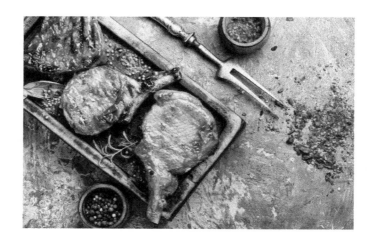

# Chili Beef

Serves: 8

Prep Time: 50 mins

Ingredients

- 3 celery ribs, finely diced

- 2 pounds grass fed beef, ground

- 2 tablespoons chili powder

- 2 tablespoons avocado oil, divided

- 2 cups grass fed beef broth

Directions

1. Heat avocado oil in a skillet on medium heat and add beef.
2. Sauté for about 3 minutes on each side and stir in broth and chili powder.
3. Cover the lid and cook for about 30 minutes on medium low heat.
4. Add celery and dish out in a bowl to serve.

Nutrition Amount per serving

Calories 223

Sodium 198mg 9%

Total Fat 11.8g 15%

Total Carbohydrate 2.4g 1%

Saturated Fat 4.7g 23%

Dietary Fiber 1.2g 4%

Cholesterol 75mg 25%

Total Sugars 0.5g

Protein 24.8g

# Smoked Brisket with Maple Syrup

Serves: 8

Prep Time: 40 mins

Ingredients

- 1 tablespoon sugar free maple syrup

- 3 pounds grass fed beef briskets

- 3 tablespoons almond oil

- 2 cups bone broth

- 4 tablespoons liquid smoke

Directions

1. Heat almond oil in a skillet on medium heat and add beef briskets.
2. Sauté for about 4 minutes per side and stir in the bone broth and liquid smoke.
3. Cover the lid and cook for about 30 minutes on medium low heat.
4. Dish out in a platter and drizzle with sugar free maple syrup to serve.

Nutrition Amount per serving

Calories    422 To-

tal Fat 17g 22%

Saturated Fat 4.9g 25%

Cholesterol 117mg 39%

Sodium 130mg 6%

Total Carbohydrate 1.7g 1%
    Dietary Fiber 0g 0% Total

    Sugars 1.5g

    Protein 61.6g

# Keto Beef Sirloin Steak

Serves: 3

Prep Time: 45 mins

Ingredients

- 3 tablespoons butter

- ½ teaspoon garlic powder

- 1 pound beef top sirloin steaks

- Salt and black pepper, to taste

- 1 garlic clove, minced

Directions

1. Heat butter in a large grill pan and add beef top sirloin steaks.
2. Brown the steaks on both sides by cooking for about 3 minutes per side.
3. Season the steaks with garlic powder, salt and black pepper and cook for about 30 minutes, flipping once.
4. Dish out the steaks to a serving platter and serve hot.

Nutrition Amount per serving

Calories   386 To-

tal Fat 21g 27%

Saturated Fat 10.9g 54%

Cholesterol 166mg 55%

Sodium 182mg 8%

Total Carbohydrate 0.7g 0%
Dietary Fiber 0.1g 0% Total

Sugars 0.1g

Protein 46.1g

# Bacon Swiss Beef Steaks

Serves: 4

Prep Time: 25 mins

Ingredients

- ½ cup Swiss cheese, shredded

- 4 beef top sirloin steaks

- 6 bacon strips, cut in half

- Salt and black pepper, to taste

- 1 tablespoon butter

Directions

1. Season the beef steaks generously with salt and black pepper.
2. Put butter in the skillet and heat on medium low heat.
3. Add beef top sirloin steaks and cook for about 5 minutes per side.
4. Add bacon strips and cook for about 15 minutes.
5. Top with Swiss cheese and cook for about 5 minutes on low heat.
6. Remove from heat and dish out on a platter to serve.

Nutrition Amount per serving

Calories 385

0.8g 0% Dietary Fiber 0g 0%

Total Fat 25.4g 33%

Saturated Fat 10.7g 54%

Sodium 552mg 24%

Cholesterol 96mg 32%

Total Sugars 0.2g Protein 35.5g

Total Carbohydrate

# Rosrmary Garlic

# Pork Chops

Preparation Time: 10 minutes Cooking Time: 35 minutes

Serve: 4

## Ingredients:

- 4 pork chops, boneless
- ¼ tsp onion powder
- 2 garlic cloves, minced
- 1 tsp dried rosemary, crushed
- ¼ tsp pepper
- ¼ tsp sea salt

## Directions:

1. Preheat the oven to 425 F.
2. Season pork chops with onion powder, pepper and salt.
3. Mix together rosemary and garlic and rub over pork chops.
4. Place pork chops on baking tray and roast for 10 minutes.
5. Set temperature 350 F and roast for 25 minutes more.
6. Serve and enjoy.

## Nutritional Value (Amount per Serving):

Calories 260

Fat 20 g

Carbohydrates 1 g

Sugar 0 g

Protein 19 g

Cholesterol 70 mg

# SOUPS, STEWS
# & SALADS

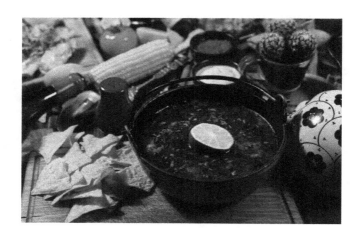

# Mushroom Chicken Soup

Preparation Time: 10 minutes Cooking Time: 20 minutes Serve: 4

## Ingredients:

- 1 tsp Italian seasoning
- 2 ½ cups chicken broth
- 1 lb chicken breast, boneless and skinless
- 1 squash, chopped
- 1 ½ cups mushrooms, chopped
- 2 garlic cloves, minced
- 1 onion, chopped
- Pepper
- Salt

## Directions:

1. Add all ingredients into the instant pot and stir well.
2. Cover slow cooker and cook on high for 15 minutes.
3. Allow to release pressure naturally then open the lid.
4. Remove chicken from pot and shred using fork.
5. Puree the soup using immersion blender.
6. Return shredded chicken to the instant pot and stir well.
7. Serve and enjoy.

**Nutritional Value (Amount per Serving):**

Calories 290

Fat 14 g

Carbohydrates 8 g

Sugar 3 g

Protein 30 g

Cholesterol 110 mg

# BRUNCH & DINNER

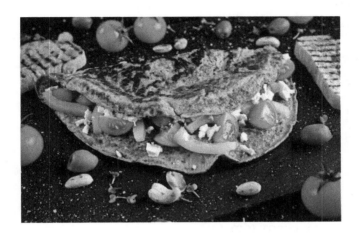

# Basil Tomato

# Frittata

Preparation Time: 10 minutes Cooking Time: 15 minutes

Serve: 2

## Ingredients:

- 5 eggs
- 1 tbsp olive oil
- 7 oz can artichokes
- 1 garlic clove, chopped
- 1 onion, chopped
- 1/2 cup cherry tomatoes
- 2 tbsp fresh basil, chopped
- 1/4 cup feta cheese, crumbled
- 1/4 tsp pepper
- 1/4 tsp salt

## Directions:

1. Heat oil in a pan over medium heat.
2. Add garlic and onion and sauté for 4 minutes.
3. Add artichokes, basil, and tomatoes and cook for 4 minutes.
4. Beat eggs in a bowl and season with pepper and salt.
5. Pour egg mixture into the pan and cook for 5-7 minutes.
6. Serve and enjoy.

## Nutritional Value (Amount per Serving):

Calories 325

Fat 22 g

Carbohydrates 14 g

Sugar 6.2 g

Protein 20 g

Cholesterol 425 mg

# DESSERTS & DRINKS

# Avocado Peanut

# Butter Fat Bombs

Preparation Time: 10 minutes Cooking Time: 10 minutes Serve: 6

### Ingredients:

- 1 tbsp swerve avocado, peeled, pitted, and chopped
- 1 cup peanut butter
- 3 tbsp heavy cream
- ½ cup butter, melted
- ½ cup coconut oil, meleted

### Directions:

➢ Add all ingredients into the blender and blend until smooth.

➢ Pour mixture into the mini cupcake liner and place in refrigerator until set.

➢ Serve and enjoy.

## Nutritional Value (Amount per Serving):

Calories 640

Fat 64 g

Carbohydrates 11 g

Sugar 4 g

Protein 11 g

Cholesterol 51 mg

# BREAKFAST RECIPES

## Chocolate Chip

## Waffles

Serves: 2

Prep Time: 30 mins

### Ingredients

- 2 scoops vanilla protein powder
- 1 pinch pink Himalayan sea salt
- 50 grams sugar free chocolate chips
- 2 large eggs, separated
- 2 tablespoons butter, melted

### Directions

1. Mix together egg yolks, vanilla protein powder and butter in a bowl.
2. Whisk together egg whites thoroughly in another bowl and transfer to the egg yolks mixture.
3. Add the sugar free chocolate chips and a pinch of pink salt.
4. Transfer this mixture in the waffle maker and cook according tomanufacturer's instructions.

## Nutrition Amount per serving

Calories  301

Total Fat 18.8g 24% Saturated Fat 9.7g 49%

Cholesterol 229mg  76%

Sodium 242mg 11%

Total Carbohydrate 6.9g 3% Dietary Fiber 1.3g

4%

Total Sugars 1.4g

# SEAFOOD RECIPES

# Roasted Trout

Serves: 4

Prep Time: 45 mins

## Ingredients

- ½ cup fresh lemon juice

- 1 pound trout fish fillets

- 4 tablespoons butter

- Salt and black pepper, to taste

- 1 teaspoon dried rosemary, crushed

## Directions

1. Put ½ pound trout fillets in a dish and sprinkle with lemon juice and dried rosemary.

2. Season with salt and black pepper and transfer into a skillet.

3. Add butter and cook, covered on medium low heat for about 35 minutes.

4. Dish out the fillets in a platter and serve with a sauce.

## Nutrition Amount per serving

Calories  349

Total Fat 28.2g 36% Saturated Fat 11.7g 58%

Cholesterol 31mg  10%

Sodium 88mg  4%

Total Carbohydrate 1.1g 0% Dietary Fiber 0.3g  1%

Total Sugars 0.9g Protein 23.3g

# APPETIZERS AND DESSERTS

# Low Carb Onion Rings

Serves: 6

Prep Time: 30 mins

### Ingredients

- 2 medium white onions, sliced into ½ inch thick rings
- ½ cup coconut flour
- 4 large eggs
- 4 oz pork rinds
- 1 cup parmesan cheese, grated

### Directions

1. Preheat an Air fryer to 3900F and grease a fryer basket.
2. Put coconut flour in one bowl, eggs in the second bowl and pork rinds and parmesan cheese in the third bowl.
3. Coat the onion rings through the three bowls one by one and repeat.
4. Place the coated onion rings in the fryer basket and cook for about 15 minutes.
5. Dish out to a platter and serve with your favorite low

carb sauce.

## Nutrition Amount per serving

Calories  270

Total Fat 15.1g 19% Saturated Fat 7.1g 35%

Cholesterol 164mg  55%

Sodium 586mg 25%

Total Carbohydrate 11g 4% Dietary Fiber 4.8g

17% Total Sugars 1.8g

Protein 24.1g

# Browned Butter

# Asparagus

Serves: 4

Prep Time: 25 mins

## Ingredients

- ½ cup sour cream
- 25 oz. green asparagus
- 3 oz. parmesan cheese, grated
- Salt and cayenne pepper, to taste
- 3 oz. butter

## Directions

1. Season the asparagus with salt and cayenne pepper.
2. Heat 1 oz. butter in a skillet over medium heat and add seasoned asparagus.
3. Sauté for about 5 minutes and dish out to a bowl.
4. Heat the rest of the butter in a skillet and cook until it is light brown and has a nutty smell.
5. Add asparagus to the butter along with sour cream and parmesan cheese.
6. Dish out to a bowl and serve hot.

## Nutrition Amount per serving

Calories 319

Total Fat 28.1g 36% Saturated Fat 17.8g 89% Cholesterol

74mg 25%

Sodium 339mg 15%

Total Carbohydrate 9.1g 3% Dietary Fiber 3.8g 14% Total

Sugars 3.4g

Protein 11.9g

# PORK AND BEEF RECIPES

## Bacon Swiss Beef Steaks

Serves: 4

Prep Time: 25 mins

### Ingredients

- ½ cup Swiss cheese, shredded
- 4 beef top sirloin steaks
- 6 bacon strips, cut in half
- Salt and black pepper, to taste
- 1 tablespoon butter

### Directions

1. Season the beef steaks generously with salt and black pepper.
2. Put butter in the skillet and heat on medium low heat.
3. Add beef top sirloin steaks and cook for about 5 minutes per side.
4. Add bacon strips and cook for about 15 minutes.
5. Top with Swiss cheese and cook for about 5 minutes on low heat.
6. Remove from heat and dish out on a platter to serve.

## Nutrition Amount per serving

Calories  385

Total Fat 25.4g 33% Saturated Fat 10.7g 54%

Cholesterol 96mg  32%

Sodium 552mg  24%

Total Carbohydrate 0.8g 0% Dietary Fiber 0g  0%

Total Sugars 0.2g Protein 35.5g

# Turkey with Mozzarella and Tomatoes

Serves: 2

Prep Time: 1 hour 30 mins

### Ingredients

- 1 tablespoon butter
- 2 large turkey breasts
- ½ cup fresh mozzarella cheese, thinly sliced
- Salt and black pepper, to taste
- 1 large Roma tomato, thinly sliced

### Directions

1. Preheat the oven to 3750F and grease the baking tray with butter.
2. Make some deep slits in the turkey breasts and season with salt and black pepper.
3. Stuff the mozzarella cheese slices and tomatoes in the turkey slits.
4. Put the stuffed turkey breasts on the baking tray and transfer to the oven.
5. Bake for about 1 hour 15 minutes and dish out to serve warm.

## Nutrition Amount per serving

Calories   104 Total Fat 7.4g  9%

Saturated Fat 4.4g 22% Cholesterol 25mg  8%

Sodium 256mg   11%

Total Carbohydrate 5.1g 2% Dietary Fiber 1g  4%

Total Sugars 2.6g Protein 5.7g

# CHICKEN AND POULTRY RECIPES

## Caprese Chicken

Serves: 4

Prep Time: 30 mins

### Ingredients

- 1 pound chicken breasts, boneless and skinless
- ¼ cup balsamic vinegar
- 1 tablespoon extra-virgin olive oil
- Kosher salt and black pepper, to taste
- 4 mozzarella cheese slices

### Directions

1. Season the chicken with salt and black pepper.
2. Heat olive oil in a skillet over medium heat and cook chicken for about 5 minutes on each side.
3. Stir in the balsamic vinegar and cook for about 2 minutes.
4. Add mozzarella cheese slices and cook for about 2 minutes until melted.
5. Dish out in a plate and serve hot.

## Nutrition Amount per serving

Calories  329

Total Fat 16.9g 22% Saturated Fat 5.8g 29%

Cholesterol 116mg  39%

Sodium 268mg   12%

Total Carbohydrate 1.1g 0% Dietary Fiber 0g  0%

Total Sugars 0.1g Protein 40.8g

## Coconut Blackberry

## Breakfast Bowl

Total Time: 10 minutes Serves: 2

**Ingredients:**

- 2 tbsp chia seeds
- ¼ cup coconut flakes
- 1 cup spinach
- ¼ cup water
- 3 tbsp ground flaxseed
- 1 cup unsweetened coconut milk
- 1 cup blackberries

**Directions:**

1. Add blackberries, flaxseed, spinach, and coconut milk into the blender and blend until smooth.
2. Fry coconut flakes in pan for 1-2 minutes.
3. Pour berry mixture into the serving bowls and sprinkle coconut flakes and chia seeds on top.
4. Serve immediately and enjoy.

**Nutritional Value (Amount per Serving): Calories 182; Fat 11.4 g; Carbohydrates 14.5 g; Sugar 4.3 g; Protein 5.3 g; Cholesterol 0 mg;**

# Chia Raspberry Pudding Shots

Total Time: 10 minutes Serves: 4

**Ingredients:**

- ½ cup raspberries
- 10 drops liquid stevia
- 1 tbsp unsweetened cocoa powder
- ¼ cup unsweetened almond milk
- ½ cup unsweetened coconut milk
- ¼ cup chia seeds

**Directions:**

Add all ingredients into the glass jar and stir well to combine.

1. Pour pudding mixture into the shot glasses and place in refrigerator for 1 hour.
2. Serve chilled and enjoy.

**Nutritional Value (Amount per Serving): Calories 117; Fat 10 g; Carbohydrates 5.9 g;**
**Sugar 1.7 g; Protein 2.7 g; Cholesterol 0mg;**

# DINNER RECIPES

# Roasted Carrots

Total Time: 45 minutes Serves: 6

**Ingredients:**

- 16 small carrots
- 1 tbsp fresh parsley, chopped
- 1 tbsp dried basil
- 6 garlic cloves, minced
- 4 tbsp olive oil
- 1 1/2 tsp salt

**Directions:**

1. Preheat the oven to 375 F/ 190 C.
2. In a bowl, combine together oil, carrots, basil, garlic, and salt.
3. Spread the carrots onto a baking tray and bake in preheated oven for 35 minutes.
4. Garnish with parsley and serve.

**Nutritional Value (Amount per Serving): Calories 139; Fat 9.4 g; Carbohydrates 14.2 g; Sugar 6.6 g; Protein 1.3 g; Cholesterol 0 mg;**

# Avocado Almond Cabbage Salad

Total Time: 15 minutes Serves: 3

**Ingredients:**

- 3 cups savoy cabbage, shredded
- ½ cup blanched almonds
- 1 avocado, chopped
- ¼ tsp pepper
- ¼ tsp sea salt
- For dressing:
- 1 tsp coconut aminos
- ½ tsp Dijon mustard
- 1 tbsp lemon juice
- 3 tbsp olive oil
- Pepper
- Salt

**Directions:**

1. In a small bowl, mix together all dressing ingredients and set aside.
2. Add all salad ingredients to the large bowl and mix well.
3. Pour dressing over salad and toss well.
4. Serve immediately and enjoy.

**Nutritional Value (Amount per Serving): Calories 317; Fat 14.1 g; Carbohydrates 39.8 g; Sugar 9.3 g; Protein 11.6 g; Cholesterol 0 mg;**

# LUNCH RECIPES

# Turnip Carrot Salad

Total Time: 50 minutes Serves: 4

**Ingredients:**

- 1 turnip, shredded
- 1/4 tsp dill
- 3 cups cabbage, shredded
- 1 carrot, shredded
- 1 green pepper, chopped
- 1 tsp salt

**Directions:**

1. Add cabbage and salt in a bowl. Cover bowl and set aside for 40 minutes.
2. Wash and cabbage and dry well.
3. Add cabbage in a bowl with remaining

   ingredients and toss well.
4. Serve and enjoy.

**Nutritional Value (Amount per Serving): Calories 34; Fat 0.1 g; Carbohydrates 7.9 g;**
**Sugar 4.3 g; Protein 1.3 g; Cholesterol 0 mg;**

# Baked Asparagus

Total Time: 25 minutes Serves: 4

**Ingredients:**

- 40 asparagus spears
- 2 tbsp vegetable seasoning
- 2 tbsp garlic powder
- 2 tbsp salt

**Directions:**

1. Preheat the oven to 450 F/ 232 C.
2. Arrange all asparagus spears on baking tray and season with vegetable seasoning, garlic powder, and salt.
3. Place in preheated oven and bake for 20 minutes.
4. Serve warm and enjoy.

**Nutritional Value (Amount per Serving): Calories 75; Fat 0.9 g; Carbohydrates 13.5 g; Sugar 5.5 g; Protein 6.7 g; Cholesterol 0 mg;**

# DESSERT RECIPES

## Avocado Pudding

Total Time: 10 minutes Serves: 8

**Ingredients:**

- 2 ripe avocados, peeled, pitted and cut into pieces
- 1 tbsp fresh lime juice
- 14 oz can coconut milk
- 80 drops of liquid stevia
- 2 tsp vanilla extract

**Directions:**

1. Add all ingredients into the blender and blend until smooth.
2. Serve and enjoy.

**Nutritional Value (Amount per Serving): Calories 317; Fat 30.1 g; Carbohydrates 9.3 g; Sugar 0.4 g; Protein 3.4 g; Cholesterol 0 mg;**

44

# BREAKFAST RECIPES

# Tuna Omelet

Breakfast would not be complete without a healthy omelet to get your day started on the right foot.

## Total Prep & Cooking Time: 15 minutes

Level: Beginner Makes: 2 Omelets

Protein: 28 grams Net Carbs: 4.9 grams

Fat: 18 grams

Sugar: 1 gram

Calories: 260

## What you need:

- 2 tbs coconut oil

- 1 medium green bell pepper, deseeded and diced

- 2 1/2 oz. canned tuna, spring water and drained

- 1/4 tsp salt

- 6 large eggs

- 1/8 tsp pepper

## Steps:

1. Melt the coconut oil in a small skillet and fry the green pepper for approximately 3 minutes. Remove from the burner.

2. Transfer the peppers into a dish and combine the tuna until fully together. Set to the side.

3. Beat the eggs, salt, and pepper in a separate dish as the coconut oil is melting in a small non-stick skillet.

4. Move the pan around to ensure the entire base is coated in oil and very hot.

5. Empty the beaten eggs into the skillet and use a rubber spatula to lift the

   edge of the cooked eggs in several areas to allow the uncooked eggs to heat.

6. Once there is a thin layer of cooked egg created, leave the pan on the heat for half a minute to fully set.

7. Scoop half of the peppers and tuna onto one side of the eggs. Use the rubber spatula to flip over the cooked eggs to create an omelet.

8. Press down lightly until the omelet naturally seals and after approximately 1 minute, move to a serving plate.

9. Repeat steps 4 through 8 with the second omelet.

*Baking Tip:*

If you do not have a ton of time in the mornings, you can create the omelet filling the evening before and refrigerate in a lidded container.

*Variation Tip:*

You may choose to garnish the top of the omelet with additional salt and pepper to taste or chopped chives.

# Radish Chips

If you are missing potato chips, these crispy radish chips might just be the ticket to your happy afternoon.

Total Prep & Cooking Time: 30 minutes

**Level: Beginner**

Makes: 4 Helpings

Protein: 1 gram Net Carbs: 2 grams Fat:

35 grams

Sugar: 2 grams

Calories: 350

**What you need:**

- 1/4 tbs onion powder

- 24 oz. extra virgin olive oil

- 1/4 tsp salt

- 48 oz. radishes, peeled & sliced

- 1/8 tsp pepper

## Steps:

1. Peel and slice the radishes to your preferred thickness.

2. In a large skillet, warm the olive oil

    then reduce the temperature.

3. Fry the radishes for approximately 40 minutes if sliced thin, up to an hour if thicker. Sprinkle with the salt, onion powder and pepper and stir occasionally.

4. Remove to a paper towel covered platter and serve.


## Baking Tip:

If you want ultra-crispy chips, slice them thin and fry for approximately 50 minutes until the edges start to curl.

# Cobb Salad

This flavorful easy to make salad can be done in advance and put into a container to bring with you to work or the gym.

Total Prep & Cooking Time: 30 minutes Level: Beginner

Makes: 1 Salad

Protein: 24 grams Net Carbs: 4.7 grams

Fat: 18 grams

Sugar: 2 grams

Calories: 337

## What you need:

- 4 cherry tomatoes

- 3/4 cup avocado

- 1 large egg

- 2 cups mixed green salad

- 1/4 cup cooked bacon, crumbled

- 2 oz. chicken breast, shredded

- 4 cups cold water

- 1 tbs coconut oil, melted

## Steps:

1. Fill a saucepan with 2 cups of the cold water and the egg.

2. Once the water starts to boil, set a timer for 7

minutes.

3. When the timer goes off, drain the water and pour the remaining 2 cups of cold water on the egg to cool.

4. Once it can be handled, peel the egg and slice into large chunks.

5. Brown the bacon in a skillet with the coconut oil until crispy. Set on a paper towel covered plate.

6. Dice the avocado and tomatoes.

7. In a bowl, empty the mixed greens and combine the chicken. Crush the bacon into the salad dish.

8. Finally, transfer the diced avocado, tomatoes and egg to the top. Serve immediately.

*Variation Tip:*

Drizzle one tablespoon of ranch dressing on top of your salad. This will add approximately

8 grams of fat and 73 calories.

# DINNER RECIPES

# Clam Chowder

This would be a wonderful dinner on a cold night and is surprisingly dairy free.

Total Prep & Cooking Time: 30 minutes Level: Beginner

Makes: 4 Helpings

Protein: 2 grams Net Carbs: 4 grams Fat:

15 grams

Sugar: 2 grams

Calories: 164

## What you need:

- 2 cups cauliflower florets
- 1 tsp onion powder
- 12 oz. steamer clams, shucked
- 1 1/3 tsp salt, separated
- 4 tbs butter, separated
- 1 1/3 cups water
- 13 oz. chicken broth
- 2 tsp rosemary
- 1/4 tsp pepper

## Steps:

1. Using a deep saucepan, dissolve 2 tablespoons of butter.

2. Heat 1 1/2 cups of the cauliflower for about 2 minutes.

3. Empty the water, onion powder, 1 tablespoon of salt, chicken broth and remaining 2 tablespoons of butter into the saucepan and heat until bubbling.

4. Bring the heat down to medium, cover the pot with a lid and let it heat for about 10 minutes.

5. Remove the saucepan from the burner and transfer to a food blender. Pulse for approximately 60 seconds until a smooth consistency.

6. Distribute the mixture back to the saucepan and combine the remaining 1/2 cup of cauliflower, 1 teaspoon of rosemary and the clams.

7. Simmer for about 10 minutes and remove from the burner.

8. Season with pepper, the remaining teaspoon of salt and the remaining teaspoon of rosemary.

## Baking Tip:

Alternatively, you can substitute ghee for the butter.

## Variation Tip:

Garnish the chowder with a tablespoon of crushed bacon to add flavoring.

# UNUSUAL DELICIOUS MEAL RECIPES

# Chicken Liver Pate

This is a traditional French dish that is loaded with healthy fats to help you liven up your Keto diet.

Total Prep & Cooking Time: 30 minutes plus 1 full day to marinate

Level: Beginner Makes: 4 Helpings

Protein: 4 grams

Net Carbs: 2.3 grams Fat: 11 grams

Sugar: 0 grams

Calories: 162

## What you need:

- 8 oz. chicken liver
- 1/2 tbs apple cider vinegar
- 3 tsp coconut oil
- 1/2 tsp rosemary, stems removed
- 8 oz. green leek, chopped
- 1/4 tsp salt
- 2 tbs balsamic vinegar
- 1/2 tsp pepper

**Steps:**

1. Marinate the chicken liver in a combination of the apple cider vinegar and water in a glass baking dish for one full day.

2. Heat a cast iron skillet until the coconut oil is dissolved.

3. Drain the livers from the marinade and transfer to the pan with the leeks, salt, and rosemary, stirring to incorporate well.

4. Place a lid on the skillet and heat for about 10 minutes. The livers will be a little pink on the inside.

5. Remove from the burner and cool for approximately 5 minutes.

6. Empty the grease and livers into a food blender, scraping the skillet with a wooden spoon to remove all contents.

7. Pulse together with the pepper and balsamic vinegar until the consistency is silky.

8. Empty into a mason jar and serve immediately. Store in the refrigerator, and it will keep up to 4 days.

# Coconut Peanut

# Butter Bars

Serves: 12

Preparation time: 10 minutes Cooking time: 10 minutes

## Ingredients:

- 1 cup unsweetened shredded coconut
- ½ tsp vanilla
- 1 tbsp swerve
- 1 cup creamy peanut butter
- ¼ cup butter
- Pinch of salt

## Directions:

- Add butter in microwave safe bowl and microwave until butter is melted.
- Add peanut butter and stir well.
- Add sweetener, vanilla, and salt and stir.
- Add shredded coconut and mix until well combined.
- Transfer mixture into the greased baking dish and spread evenly.

- Place in refrigerator for 1 hour.

- Slice and serve.

Per Serving: Net Carbs: 3.8g; Calories: 221 Total Fat: 20g; Saturated Fat: 9.4g Protein: 6.1g; Carbs: 6.4g; Fiber: 2.6g; Sugar: 2.7g; Fat 82% / Protein 12% / Carbs 6

# CAKE

## Delicious Almond

## Apple Tart

Serves: 10

Preparation time: 10 minutes Cooking time: 55 minutes

*For crust:*

- 2 cups almond flour
- 6 tbsp butter, melted
- 1/2 tsp cinnamon
- 1/3 cup erythritol

*For filling:*

- 1/4 cup erythritol
- 3 cups apples, peeled, cored, and sliced
- 1/2 tsp cinnamon
- 1/4 cup butter
- 1/2 tsp lemon juice

**Directions:**

1. Preheat the oven to 375 F/ 190 C.
2. For the crust: In a bowl, mix together butter, cinnamon, swerve, and almond flour until it looks crumbly.
3. Transfer crust mixture into the 10- inch spring-form

pan and spread evenly using your fingers.

4. Bake crust in preheated oven for 5 minutes.

5. For the filling: In a bowl, mix together apple slices and lemon juice.

6. Arrange apple slices evenly across the bottom of the baked crust in a circular shape.

7. Press apple slices down lightly.

8. In a small bowl, combine together butter, swerve, and cinnamon and microwave for 1 minute.

9. Whisk until smooth and pour over apple slices.

10. Bake tart for 30 minutes.

11. Remove from oven and lightly press down apple slices with a fork.

12. Turn heat to 350 F/ 180 C and bake for 20 minutes more.

13. Remove from the oven and set aside to cool completely.

14. Slice and serve.

Per Serving: Net Carbs: 3.7g; Calories: 236; Total Fat: 22.7g; Saturated Fat: 8.1g

Protein: 5g; Carbs: 6.4g; Fiber: 2.7g; Sugar: 1.9g; Fat 86% / Protein 8% / Carbs 6%

# Cake

Serves: 16

Preparation time: 10 minutes Cooking time: 40 minutes

## Ingredients:

- 4 eggs
- 1 tsp baking powder
- 1 1/2 tsp vanilla
- 1/3 cup Swerve
- 2 oz cream cheese, softened
- 2 tbsp butter
- 1 cup almond flour
- 1/2 cup coconut flour
- 4 oz half and half
- Pinch of salt
- For topping:
- 3/4 cup almonds, toasted and sliced
- 1/3 cup Swerve
- 6 tbsp butter, melted
- 1 cup almond flour

## Directions:

1. Preheat the oven to 350 F/ 180 C.
2. Spray 8-inch cake pan with cooking spray and set aside.
3. Add all ingredients except topping ingredients into the large

85

bowl whisk until well combined.

4.  Pour batter into the prepared cake pan and spread evenly.

5.  Combine together all topping ingredients.

6.  Sprinkle topping mixture evenly on top of batter.

7.  Bake for 40 minutes.

8.  Remove from oven and allow to cool completely.

9.  Slice and serve.

Per Serving: Net Carbs: 2.8g; Calories: 198 Total Fat: 18.2g; Saturated Fat: 6g

Protein: 5.9g; Carbs: 5g; Fiber: 2.2g; Sugar: 0.9g; Fat 83% / Protein 12% / Carbs 5%

# Cocoa Butter Candy

Serves: 8

Preparation time: 5 minutes Cooking time: 5

minutes

## Ingredients:

- 1/4 cup cocoa butter
- 10 drops stevia
- 1/4 cup coconut oil

## Directions:

1. Melt together coconut oil and cocoa butter in a saucepan over low heat.
2. Remove from heat and stir in stevia.
3. Pour mixture into the silicone candy mold and refrigerate until hardened.
4. Serve and enjoy.

Per Serving: Net Carbs: 0g; Calories: 119; Total Fat: 13.8g; Saturated Fat: 9.9g

Protein: 0g; Carbs: 0g; Fiber: 0g; Sugar: 0g; Fat 100% / Protein 0% / Carbs 0%

# FROZEN DESSERT: BEGINNER

## Strawberry Ice Cream

Serves: 4

Preparation time: 5 minutes Cooking time: 10 minutes

**Ingredients:**

- 2 tbsp sour cream
- 1/3 cup Swerve
- ½ cup strawberries, sliced
- 2 cups heavy cream
- ½ tsp vanilla

**Directions:**

1. Add all ingredients into the blender and blend until smooth.
2. Pour mixture into a metal loaf pan and place in the refrigerator for 5-6 hours.
3. Defrost ice cream for 20 minutes until soft.
4. Serve and enjoy.

Per Serving: Net Carbs: 3.2g; Calories: 228; Total Fat: 23.5g; Saturated Fat: 14.6g

Protein: 1.5g; Carbs: 3.6g; Fiber: 0.4g; Sugar: 1g; Fat 93% / Protein 2% / Carbs 5%

# COOKIES: BEGINNER

## Gingersnap Cookies

Serves: 8

Preparation time: 10 minutes Cooking time: 10 minutes

### Ingredients:

- 1 egg
- ½ tsp vanilla
- 1/8 tsp ground cloves
- ¼ tsp ground nutmeg
- ¼ tsp ground cinnamon
- ½ tsp ground ginger
- 1 tsp baking powder
- ¾ cup erythritol
- 2/4 cup butter, melted
- 1 ½ cups almond flour
- Pinch of salt

### Directions:

1. In a mixing bowl, mix together all dry ingredients.
2. In another bowl, mix together all wet ingredients.
3. Add dry ingredients to the wet ingredients and mix until dough-like mixture is formed.

4. Cover and place in the refrigerator for 30 minutes.

5. Preheat the oven to 350 F/ 180 C.

6. Line baking tray with parchment paper and set aside.

7. Make cookies from dough and place on a prepared baking tray.

8. Bake in for 10-15 minutes.

9. Serve and enjoy.

Per Serving: Net Carbs: 2.8g; Calories: 232; Total Fat: 22.6g; Saturated Fat: 8.2g

Protein: 5.3g; Carbs: 5.1g; Fiber: 2.3g; Sugar: 0.8g; Fat 87% / Protein 9% / Carbs 4%

# Intermediate: Creamy Raspberry Cheesecake Ice Cream

Serves: 8

Preparation time: 10 minutes Cooking time: 30 minutes

## Ingredients:

- 1 tbsp swerve
- 4 oz raspberries
- 1 tsp vanilla
- ½ cup unsweetened almond milk
- 1 ½ cups heavy cream
- ¾ cup Swerve
- 8 oz cream cheese, softened

## Directions:

1. In a large bowl, beat together cream cheese and swerve until smooth.
2. Add vanilla, almond milk, and heavy cream and mix

well.

3. Pour ice cream mixture into the ice cream maker and churn according to machine instructions.

4. In a small bowl, mash raspberries. Add 1 tbsp swerve in mashed raspberries and mix well.

5. Add mash raspberry mixture to the ice cream.

6. Serve and enjoy.

Per Serving: Net Carbs: 2.5g; Calories: 188 Total Fat: 18.5g; Saturated Fat: 11.4g

Protein: 2.8g; Carbs: 3.5g; Fiber: 1g; Sugar: 0.8g; Fat 89% / Protein 6% / Carbs 5%

# BREAKFAST RECIPES

## Convenient Hiking Sandwich

All out: 15 min Prep: 15 min

Yield: 4 servings

**Ingredients**

- 1 round portion nation style dry bread (around 1 pound)
- 1/2 cup pesto sauce (acquired or natively constructed)
- 1/2 pound meagerly cut prosciutto, top-quality ham, or smoked turkey
- 1/2 pound meagerly cut Parrano cheddar, Monterey Jack, or provolone
- 2 enormous red ringer peppers, simmered, stripped and cut into wide strips; or 1 container broiled
- red chime peppers
- 2 ready tomatoes, cut

**Direction**

1. Spot the portion of bread on a board and with a sharp blade, cut a huge hover in the highest point of the bread, around 1-inch in from the edge, making a cover.

Evacuate cover and haul out internal parts of bread from both base and top, making a bread shell. (Save hauled out bread for breadcrumbs or to encourage the winged creatures!). Spread around 2/3 of the pesto sauce over within the bread base, covering as uniformly as could be expected under the circumstances. Spread the rest of the pesto on the underside of the bread cover. Layer 1/3 of the cut meat in the base of the bread base, tucking it into the sides. Top with 1/2 of the cut cheddar, at that point 1/2 of the peppers, at that point a large portion of the tomato cuts. Rehash layers, finishing with the last 1/3 of the meat on top. Make sure to fold meat, cheddar, and vegetables into the sides of the bread base just as in the inside.

2.  Supplant the bread top so it lines up with the cut imprints. Enclose the sandwich by plastic or a handkerchief, fixing firmly. Use a sharp blade into 4 wedges and serve.

# Roasted Herb

# Crackers

Servings: 75 crackers

Nutritional Values:

**Calories: 34, Total Fat: 5.1 g, Saturated Fat: 0.3 g,**

**Carbs: 1.5 g, Sugars: 0.3 g,**

**Protein: 1.3 g Ingredients:**

- ¼ cup Avocado Oil
- 10 Celery Stalks
- 1 sprig Fresh Rosemary, stem discarded
- 2 sprigs Fresh Thyme, stems discarded
- 2 Tbsp Apple Cider Vinegar
- 1 tsp Himalayan Salt
- 3 cups Ground Flax Seed

**Directions:**

1. Preheat your oven to 225F / 110C.

2. Add the oil, celery, herbs, vinegar, and salt to your food processor and pulse until pureed. Add the flax and pulse again to incorporate and let sit for about 2-3 minutes until the mixture firms up.

3. Bake in the preheated oven for about an hour. Remove the parchment paper, flip the crackers and bake for one

more hour. If the crackers are thick, they will need more time to bake.

4.  Let it cool before serving.

# Keto Rosemary Rolls

Cooking time: 20 min

Yield : 8 rolls

**Nutrition facts: 89 calories per roll: Carbs 2.3g, fats 7.7g, and 3.3g proteins.**

**Ingredients:**

- 2 tsp fresh rosemary
- 1 tbsp baking powder
- 4 oz cream cheese
- 3/4 cup mozzarella cheese, shredded
- 1 tsp dried chives
- 1 egg
- 1 cup almond flour

**Steps:**

1. Heat oven to 160°C.
2. Mix all dry ingredients: almond flour+baking powder+dried chives+fresh rosemary.
3. Microwave mozzarella+cream cheese for a minute.
4. Add there an egg and mix again.
5. Add to the egg with cheese mixed dry ingredients and make the dough.
6. Let it cool in a freezer for 15 min.

7. Oil your hands and form 8 small balls

8. Put them on a baking tray covered with the butter paper.

Bake for 20 min.

# SNACKS RECIPES

## Intermediate: Nuts bread

Servings: 10-12

Cooking time: 75 minutes

**Nutrients per one serving: Calories: 103 | Fats: 13.1 g | Carbs: 1.6 g | Proteins: 6.5 g**

**Ingredients:**

- 1 cup almond flour
- 3 eggs
- ¼ cup olive oil
- 2 oz Brazil nuts
- 2 oz hazelnuts
- 2 oz walnuts
- ½ cup sesame seeds
- 2 tbsp flax seeds
- 2 tbsp pumpkin seeds
- A pinch of salt

**Cooking process:**

1. The oven to be preheated to 170°C (338°F).

2. Crush all the nuts in a blender until uniformity.

3. In a bowl, mix the dry ingredients. Add whipped eggs and butter. Mix it all.

4. Grease the baking dish. Lay out the dough. Bake in the oven for 60 minutes.

# Keto Mug Bread

Preparation Time: 2 min Cooking Time: 2
min

Servings:1

**Nutritional Values:**

Fat: 37 g.

Protein: 15 g.

Carbs: 8 g.

## Ingredients:

- 1/3 cup Almond Flour
- ½ tsp Baking Powder
- ¼ tsp Salt
- 1 Whole Egg
- 1 tbsp Melted Butter

## Directions:

1. Mix all ingredients in a microwave- safe mug.
2. Microwave for 90 seconds.
3. Cool for 2 minutes.
4. Keto Blender Buns

# DINNER

## Chili Crackers

Servings:30 crackers

Nutritional Values: Calories: 49, Total Fat: 4.1 g, Saturated Fat: 1.2 g, Carbs: 2.8 g, Sugars: 0.1 g, Protein: 1.6 g

### Ingredients:

- ¾ cup Almond Flour
- ¼ cup Coconut Flour
- ¼ cup Flax Seed
- ½ tsp Paprika
- ½ tsp Cumin
- 1 1/2 tsp Chili Pepper Spice
- 1 tsp Onion Powder
- ½ tsp Salt
- 1 Egg
- ¼ cup Unsalted Butter

**Directions:**

1. Preheat your oven to 350F / 175C.

2. Pulse the ingredients until dough forms.

3. Divide the dough into two equal parts. Cut into crackers and repeat the same with the other ball of dough. Transfer the crackers to the prepared baking tray.

4. Bake for about 8-10 minutes. When done, remove from the oven, leave to cool and serve.

# Thursday:

# Breakfast:

# Friday: Breakfast:

# Break the Fast

# Burrito Bowl

Skip the carbs from the tortilla by putting leftover seasoned beef and veggies into a bowl. So easy.

Variation tip: try different toppings, like salsa. Prep Time: 5 minutes

Cook Time: 15 minutes

Serves 2

**What's in it**

- Seasoned ground beef – can use Keto Taco recipe (.5 pounds)
- Prepared riced cauliflower (2 cups)
- Chopped cilantro (2 T)
- Butter (2 t, divided)
- Eggs (3 qty)
- Salt (to taste)
- Pepper (to taste)

**How it's made**

1. Brown and season the beef in a large skillet with a teaspoon of the butter. When done, push to one side.

2. Add diced cauliflower and chopped cilantro. Season with salt. Push to the side.

3. Melt a teaspoon of butter in the open space of the skillet.

4. Beat the eggs and add to the butter. Scramble in the skillet. If your skillet isn't large enough for this step, use a separate pan.

5. Mix everything together. Taste.

6. Season with salt and pepper if necessary.

**Net carbs: 4 grams**

Fat: 14 grams

Protein: 34 grams

Sugars: 2 grams

# Pancakes, The Keto Way

What a treat! Pancakes on the keto diet. If you thought you would miss fluffy pancakes, then try these. They're delicious.

Variation tip: serve with berries and homemade whipped cream, peanut butter or even crumpled, crispy bacon.

Prep Time: 5 minutes Cook Time: 10 minutes Serves 4

## What's in it

- Eggs (4 qty)
- Cottage cheese (7 ounces)
- Ground psyllium husk powder (At healthy grocery stores 1T)
- Butter (2 ounces)

## How it's made

1. Mix eggs, cheese and psyllium husk powder together and set aside. The mixture will thicken.

2. Over medium heat, melt butter in a nonstick skillet. When melted and slightly bubbly, pour 3 T of pancake batter and cook for 4 minutes. Flip and cook for 3 more minutes. Proceed with the rest of the batter.

## Net carbs: 5 grams

Fat: 39 grams

Protein: 13 grams; Sugars: 2 grams

# Wednesday: Dinner:

# Keto Tacos

Tacos get a makeover too. Instead of tortillas, filling is stuffed into zucchini boats. Make extra seasoning to always have on hand for taco meat anytime.

Variation tips: Try different types of cheeses. Serve with salsa.

Prep Time: 15 minutes Cook Time: 30 minutes

Serves 4

**What's in it**

- Zucchini (2 qty)

- Extra virgin olive oil (3 T, divided)

- Grass fed ground beef or pork (1 pound)

- Kosher salt (1 t)

- White onion, chopped (.25 cup)

- Chili powder (1 t)

- Cumin (.5 t)

- Oregano (.5 t)

- Shredded cheddar cheese (1.25 cups)

**How it's made**

1. Turn oven to 400 degrees F to preheat.

2. Slice zucchini in half lengthwise and scoop out seeds to

make boats. Sprinkle with kosher salt. Let sit for about 10 minutes.

3. Heat 2 T of extra virgin olive oil in skillet and brown meat.

4. Add chili powder, cumin, oregano and salt. Cook until liquid is mostly gone.

5. Blot zucchini with a paper towel and put on a baking sheet that has been greased.

6. Mix 1/3 of cheese in the seasoned beef.

7. Stuff the cheesy beef into the zucchini boats evenly and place in hot oven for about 20 minutes until cheese starts to turn brown. Remove from the oven and let cool for a few minutes.

**Net carbs: 6 grams**

Fat: 49 grams

Protein: 33 grams

Sugars: 2 grams

# Thursday: Dinner: On the go chicken wings with green beans

We decided to incorporate a meal idea here to illustrate how you can build your keto meals when you're pressed for time.

**What's In it:**

- Pecan smoked chicken wings (frozen, available at WalMart)
- Marketside French Green beans (fresh and packaged for microwaving, available at Walmart.
- How it's made:
- Preheat oven to 425.
- Bake chicken wings for 30-35 minutes.
- When chicken wings are almost done, place beans inside a microwave in the bag and cook for 2-3 minutes.
- Take beans out and season with butter or olive oil, and salt and pepper.
- Enjoy with your chicken wings!

**Net carbs: 7 grams**

1. Fat: 14 grams per 4 ounces serving of chicken, be sure to add butter or olive oil used

2. Protein: 14 grams per 4 ounces serving of chicken

3. Sugars: 3 grams

CPSIA information can be obtained
at www.ICGtesting.com
Printed in the USA
BVHW091130230221
600894BV00003B/320